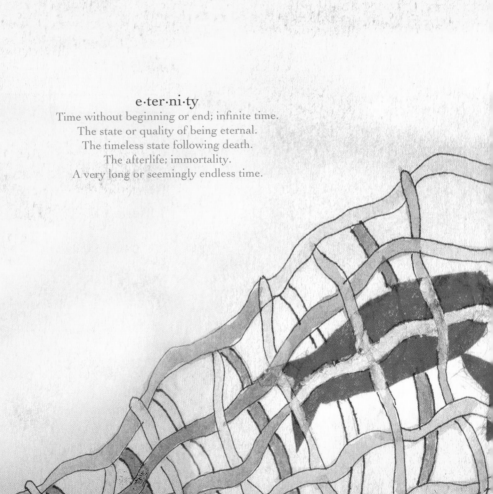

e·ter·ni·ty
Time without beginning or end; infinite time.
The state or quality of being eternal.
The timeless state following death.
The afterlife; immortality.
A very long or seemingly endless time.

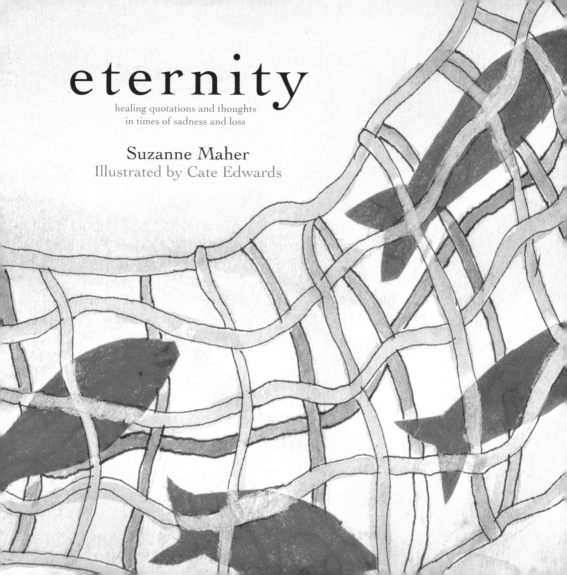

eternity

healing quotations and thoughts
in times of sadness and loss

Suzanne Maher
Illustrated by Cate Edwards

Selection and design by Suzanne Maher.

Edited by Barbara Maher.

First published in 2006 by Affirmations Australia Pty Ltd.

07 08 09 10 11 WKT 10 9 8 7 6 5 4 3 2 1

ISBN-13: 978-0-7407-6914-6
ISBN-10: 0-7407-6914-6

Library of Congress Control Number: 2007922165

www.andrewsmcmeel.com

Attention: Schools and Businesses
Andrews McMeel books are available at quantity discounts with bulk purchase for educational, business, or sales promotional use. For information, please write to: Special Sales Department, Andrews McMeel Publishing, LLC, 4520 Main Street, Kansas City, Missouri 64111.

All Elisabeth Kübler-Ross quotations have been selected from
The Wheel of Life by Dr. Elisabeth Kübler-Ross, published by Bantam Press.
Reprinted by permission of the Random House Group Ltd.
and Dr. Elisabeth Kübler-Ross's Web sites,
www.elisabethkublerross.com and www.ekrfoundation.org.

Every effort has been made to acknowledge the author of the quotations used.
Please contact the publisher if this has not occurred.

For Carol, my twin sister and soul mate,

and to Cath,
whose spirit entered my heart and has never left.

let us begin the journey home

Deepest thanks to those who have unknowingly inspired me and contributed to the creation of this book.
To Cate, an incredible channel of creativity, you never cease to delight me with your art,
and to Barb, for your imaginative help.

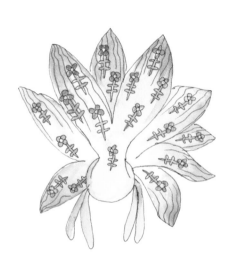

what if you slept
and what if in your sleep you dreamed
and what if in your dream you went to heaven
and there you plucked a strange and beautiful flower
and what if when you awoke
you had the flower in your hand?

oh, what then?

samuel taylor coleridge

the spiritual journey
is individual

highly personal

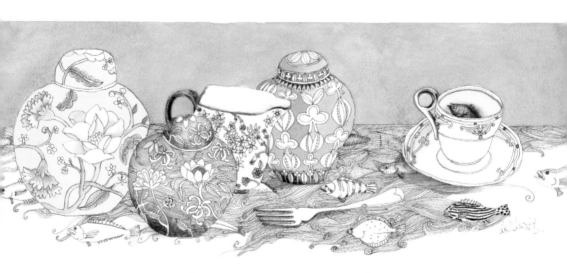

listen to your own truth

hold
tenderly

that which you cherish

savor self sweet spirit silence succumb

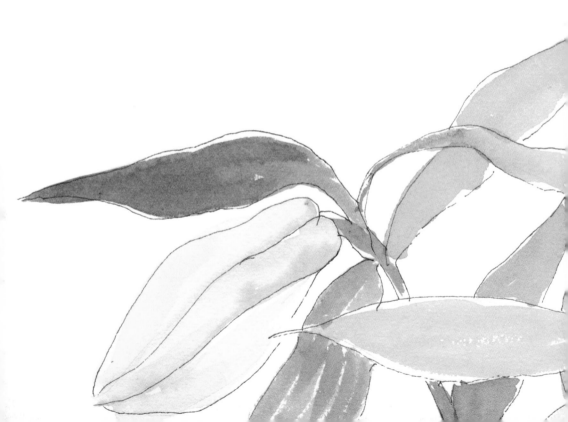

simplicity search soul surrender serenity

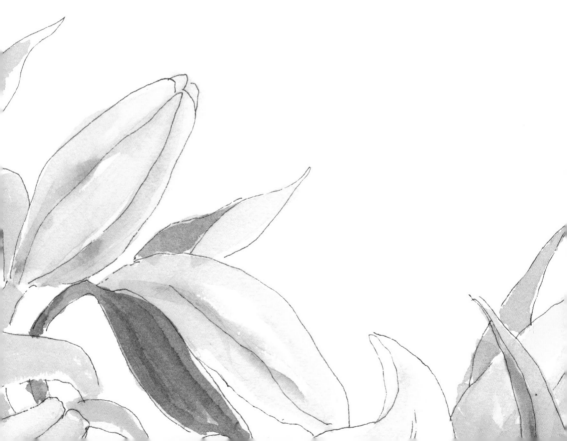

take time to laugh

it is the music
of the soul

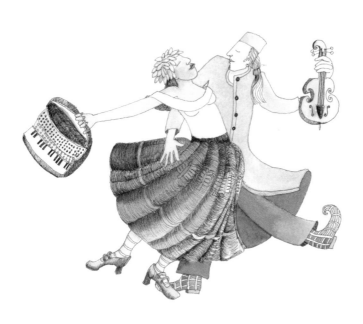

be kind
everyone you meet is fighting a hard battle

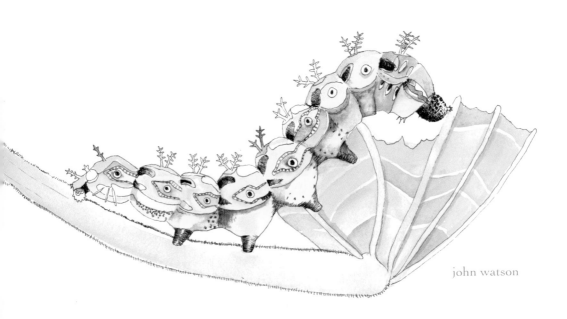

john watson

the bitterest tears

shed over graves

are for words

left unsaid

and deeds left undone

harriet beecher stowe

you must love with your time your hands and your hearts

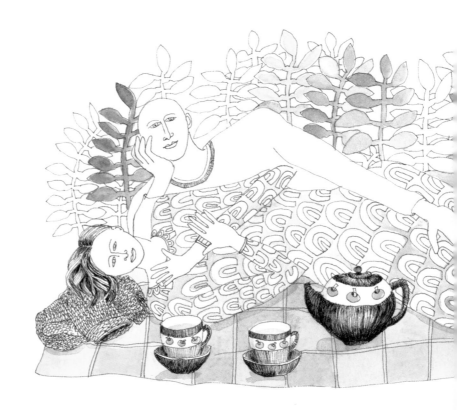

you need to share all that you have

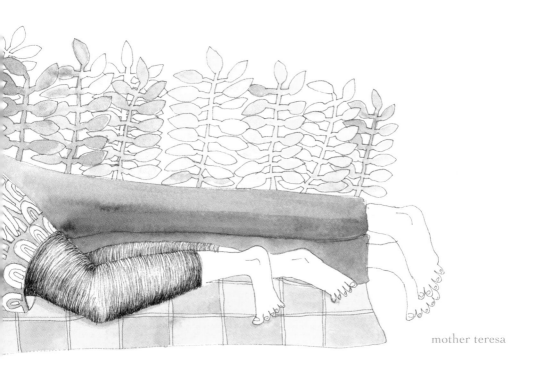

mother teresa

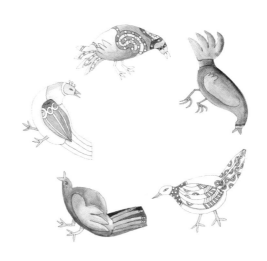

do not take life's
experiences too seriously

above all do not let them hurt you
for in reality they are nothing
but dream experiences

if circumstances are bad
and you have to bear them
do not make them
a part of yourself

play your part in life
but never forget
that it is only a role

paramahansa yogananda

not everything
that can be counted
counts
and
not everything that counts
can be counted

albert einstein

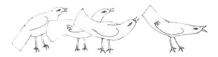

the more the marble wastes
the more the statue grows

michelangelo

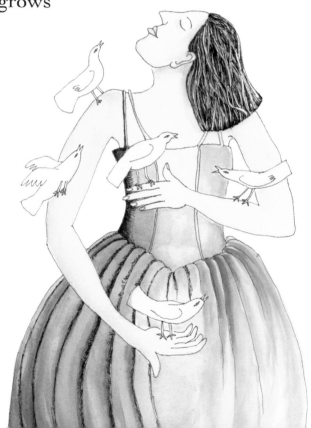

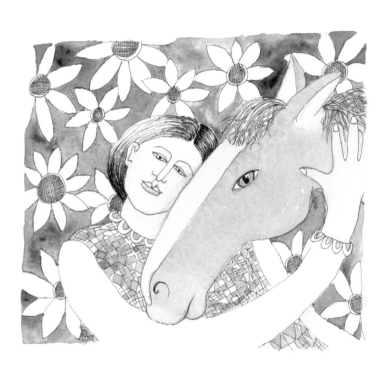

when the student is ready
the master appears

buddhist proverb

it is only with the heart that one can see rightly

antoine de saint-exupéry

those whom true love has held
it will go on holding

lucius annaeus seneca

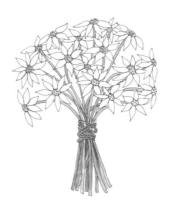

there are two days
in a week
about which and upon which
to never worry

one of these days is yesterday
and the other day
is tomorrow

robert jones burdette

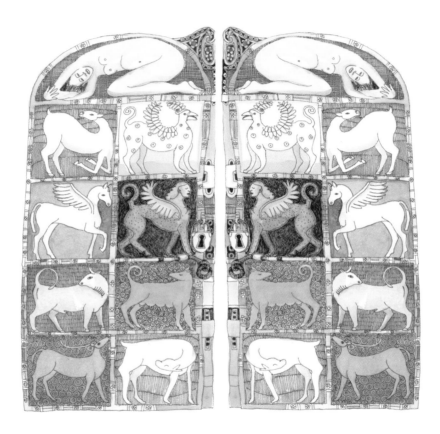

trust in dreams

for in them
is hidden
the gate to eternity

kahlil gibran

the pain goes away

all things grow with time
except grief

jewish proverb

everyone
goes through hardship in life

the more you go through
the more you learn and grow

elisabeth kübler-ross

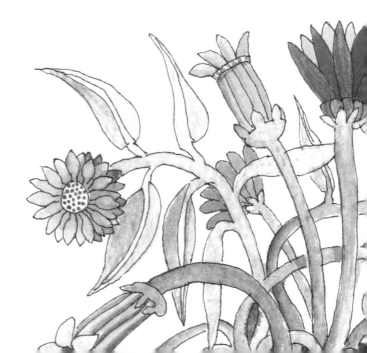

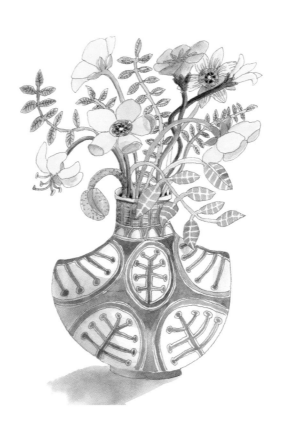

hold on to what is good
even if it is a handful of earth

hold on to what you believe
even if it is a tree
which stands by itself

hold on to what you must do
even if it is
a long way from here

hold on to life
even when it is easier to let go
and

hold on to my hand
even when
i have gone away from you

pueblo verse

retreat

refresh

remember

respect

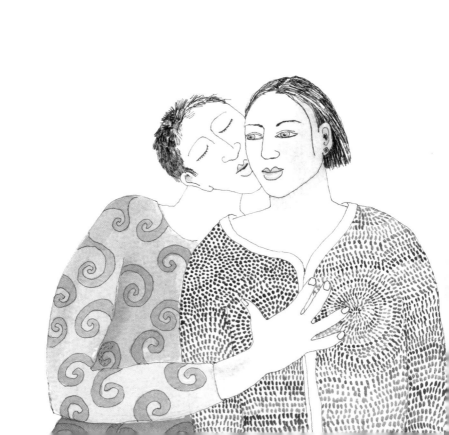

think of all the beauty still left around you
and
be happy

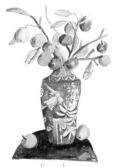

anne frank

do not squander today
for there may be
no tomorrow

tibetan motto

death is but a transition
from this life
to another existence

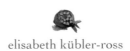

elisabeth kübler-ross

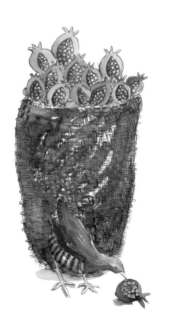

you must understand
the whole of life

not just one little part of it

that is why you must read
that is why you must look at the skies
that is why you must sing and dance
and write poems
and suffer and understand
for that is life

jiddu krishnamurti

open
your
heart
and
let the wellsprings flow

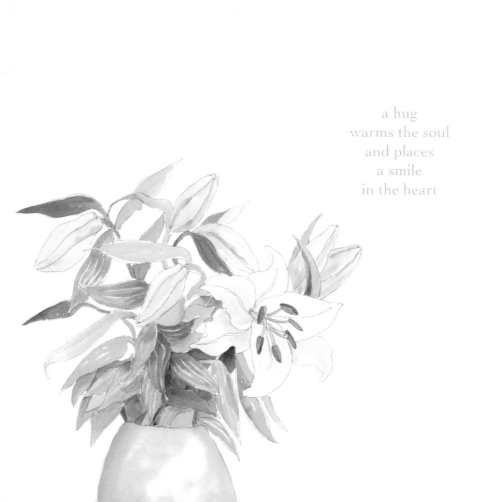

a hug
warms the soul
and places
a smile
in the heart

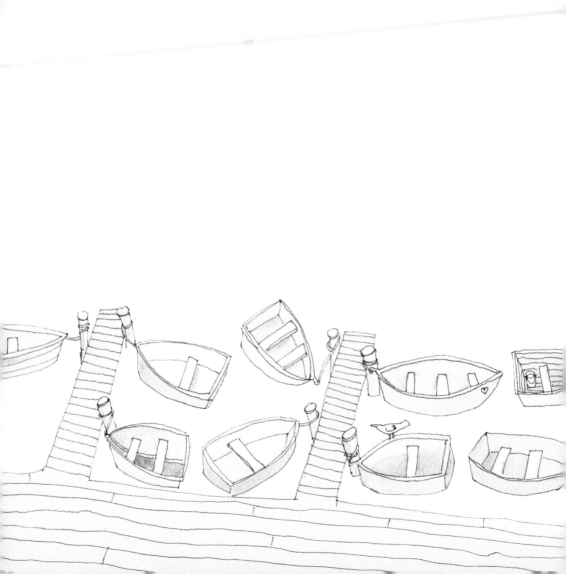

gentle time
will heal our sorrows

sophocles

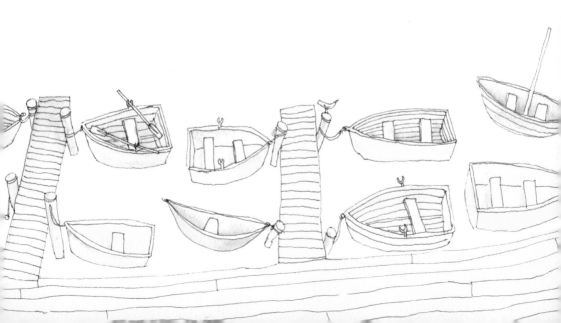

life is a journey
we are all passengers
on a boat called life
and we are all alive in the moment called now

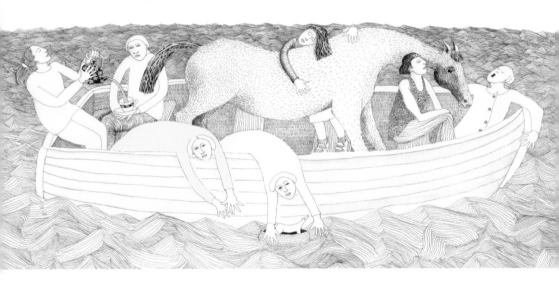

the journey of life is so beautiful
that it needs no destination

be
swift
to
love
and
make
haste
to
be
kind

henri frédéric amiel

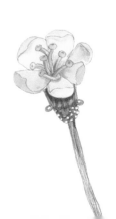

in heaven
an angel
is nobody in particular

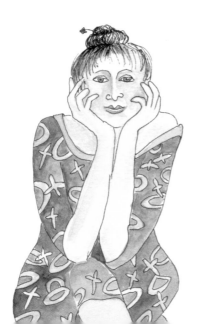

three things in human life
are important

the first is to be kind
the second is to be kind
and the third

is to be kind

henry james

the reality of life is life itself
whose beginning is not in the womb
and whose ending is not in the grave

for the years that pass
are naught but a moment
in eternal life
and the world of matter
and all in it
is but a dream

kahlil gibran

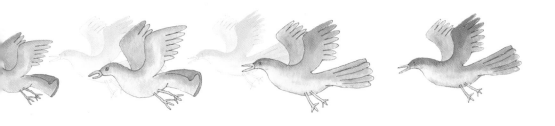

life is a voyage that is homeward bound

herman melville

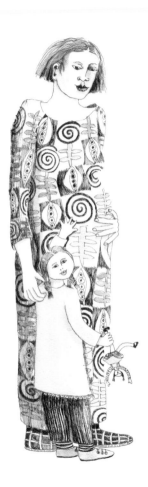

forgive
everyone
everything
every day

there is only one path to heaven
on earth we call it

risk reopen reconstruct relax release

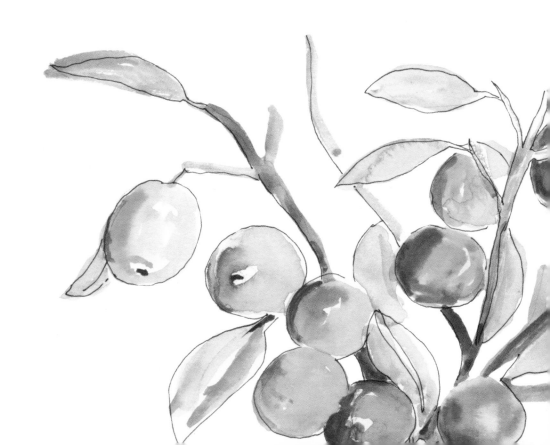

refresh rethink reveal regard remember

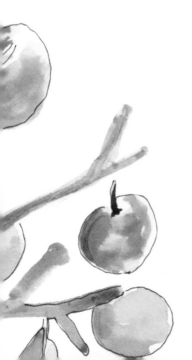

never shall i forget the time
i spent with you

please continue to be my friend
as you will always find me yours

ludwig van beethoven

he turns
not back
who is
bound
to a
star

leonardo da vinci

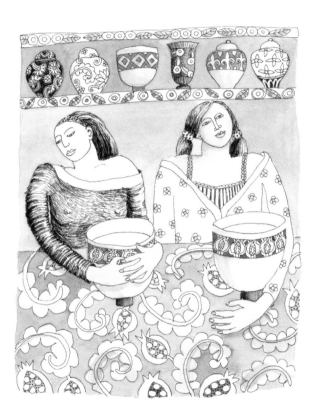

the most beautiful people
we have known
are those
who have known defeat
known suffering
known struggle
known loss

and have found their way
out of the depths

beautiful people do not just happen

elisabeth kübler-ross

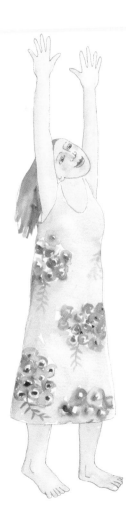

heaven is under our feet
as well as over our heads

henry david thoreau

a little while

forget not
that i shall come back to you

a little while
and my longing shall gather
dust and foam for another body

a little while
a moment of rest upon the wind

kahlil gibran

discover that you have two hands

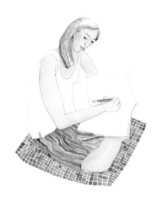

one for helping yourself
the other for helping others

abraham lincoln

you
can
never
do
a
kindness
too
soon
because
you
never
know
how
soon
it
will
be
too late

ralph waldo emerson

be yourself

there is no one better qualified

we are each gifted
in a unique
and important way

it is our privilege
and our adventure
to discover
our own special light

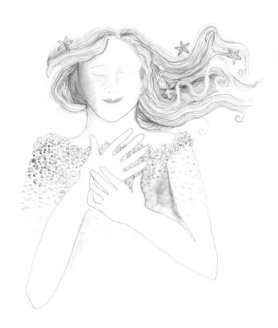

mary dunbar

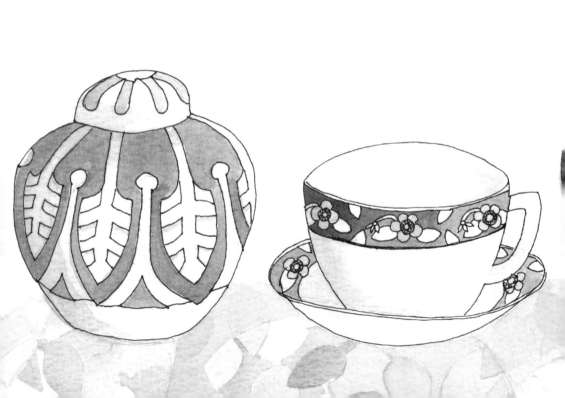

it is hard to find a being of great wisdom

rare are the places in which they are born

those who accompany them
when they appear
know good fortune indeed

dhammapada - 193

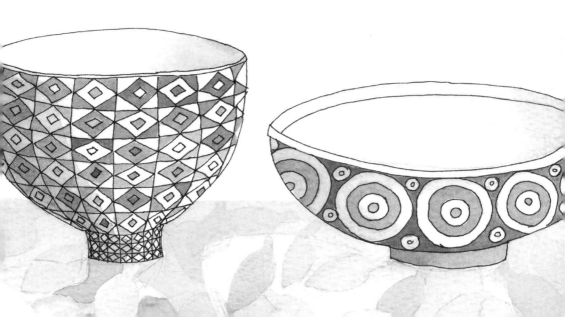

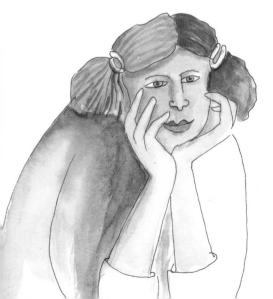

life is
just a chance
to grow
a soul

a powell davies

italian proverb

once the game is over
the king and pawn
go into the same box

each small part
of everyday life
is part of the total harmony
of the universe

st thérèse de lisieux

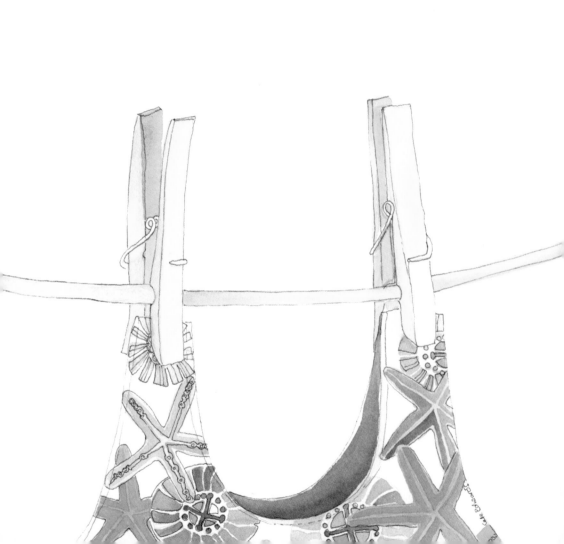

for
everything
there
is a
season
and a
time
for
every
matter
under
heaven

ecclesiastes 3:1

the only thing
that lives forever
is love

elisabeth kübler-ross

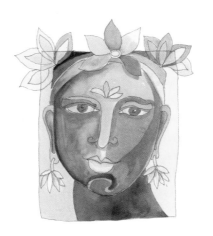

my message to you is this

be courageous
have faith
go forward

thomas edison

when you are sorrowful
look in your heart
and you shall see
that in truth
you are weeping
for that which has been
your delight

kahlil gibran

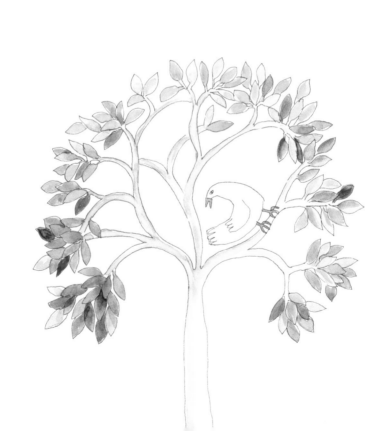

nobody

can give you

wiser advice

than

yourself

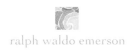

ralph waldo emerson

when once you have tasted flight
  you will forever walk the earth
  with your eyes turned skyward

                            for there you have been
                            and there you will always
                            long to return

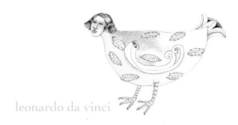

leonardo da vinci

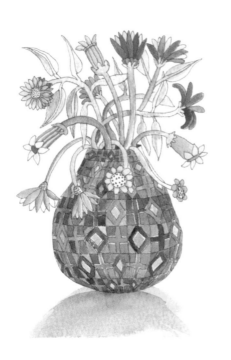

flowers
feed
the
soul

muhammad

stillness is the altar of spirit

paramahansa yogananda

the
best
thing
about
the
future
is
that
it
only
comes
one
day
at
a
time

abraham lincoln

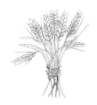

we feel and know that we are eternal

baruch spinoza

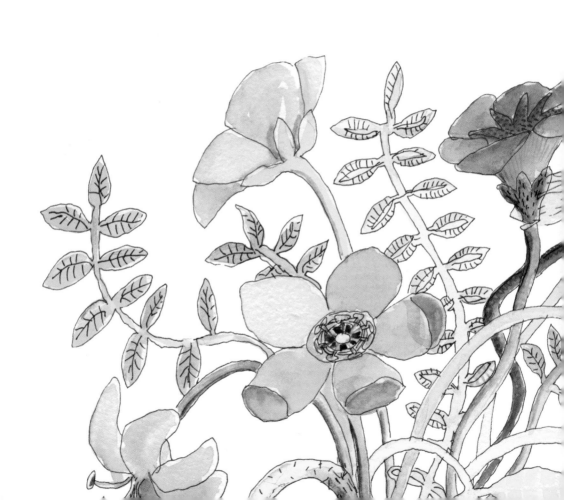

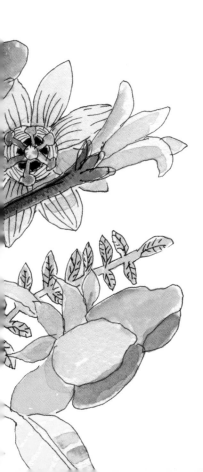

from
the
instant
our
souls
met
our
souls
flowered

oscar wilde

let your soul smile
through your heart
and your heart smile
through your eyes
that you may scatter rich smiles
in sad hearts

paramahansa yogananda

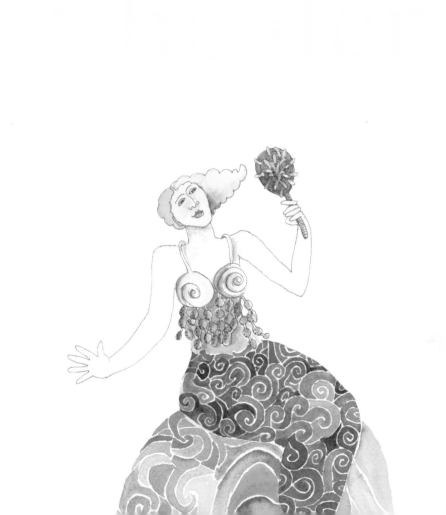

our

grief

is as

individual

as our

lives

elisabeth kübler-ross

live for those
who love you
for those who know you true
for the heaven that smiles above you
and awaits your coming too

for the cause that lacks resistance
for the future and the distance
and
all the good that you can do

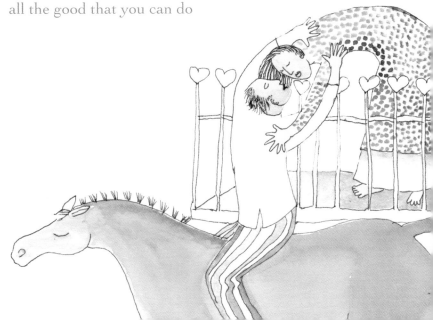

beyond this world and life we know there is someone watching over us

rumi

listen now
to the gentle whispers

be grateful for whatever comes

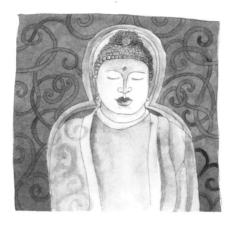

because each has been sent as a guide from beyond

rumi

desire

ask

believe

receive

we are all a part of
the same great body
the beat
our beat
unifies our hearts
and our spirits
with love and light

listen
feel
and celebrate the connection

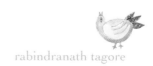

rabindranath tagore

the Divine
became the father
to love you through wisdom
and
became the mother
to give you unconditional love

paramahansa yogananda

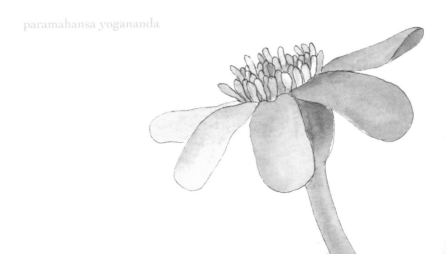

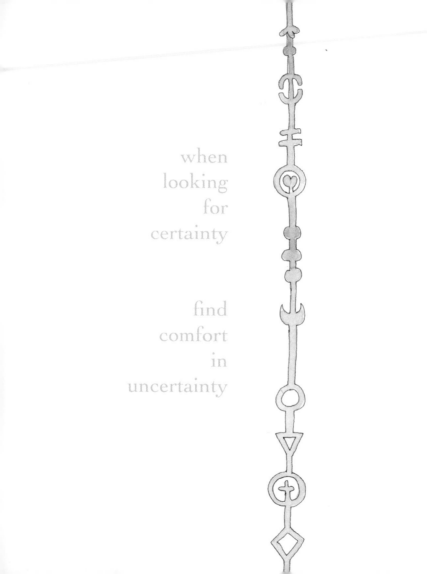

when
looking
for
certainty

find
comfort
in
uncertainty

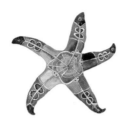

isn't it comforting to know that we are a part
of something truly miraculous

rabindranath tagore

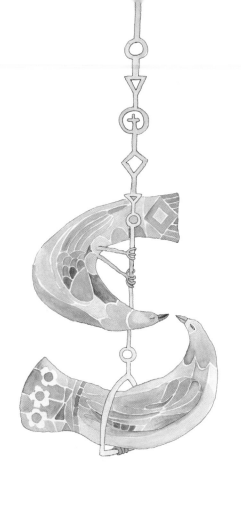

one day your heart
will take you to your lover

one day your soul
will carry you to the Beloved

don't get lost in your pain

know that one day
your pain will become your cure

rumi

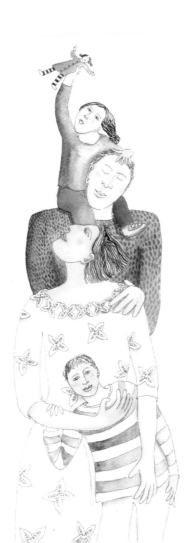

home is where
the heart can laugh
without shyness

home is where
the heart's tears
can dry
at their own pace

vernon baker

let no one
ever come to you
without leaving
better
and happier

mother teresa

but oh for the touch of a vanished hand
and the sound of a voice that is still

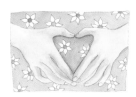

alfred lord tennyson

there is within each of us
a potential for goodness
beyond our imagining

for giving which seeks no reward

for listening without judgment

for loving unconditionally

elisabeth kübler-ross

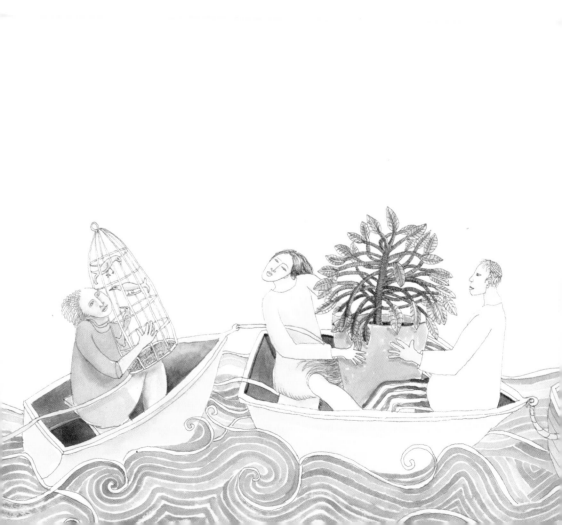

leave a legacy for future generations

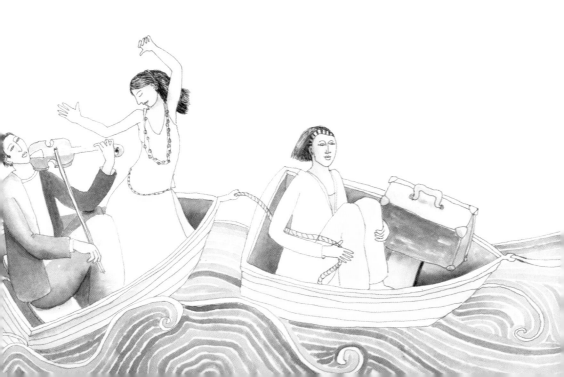

there are moments
in which one
is so completely alone

jules renaud

patience
is the companion of wisdom

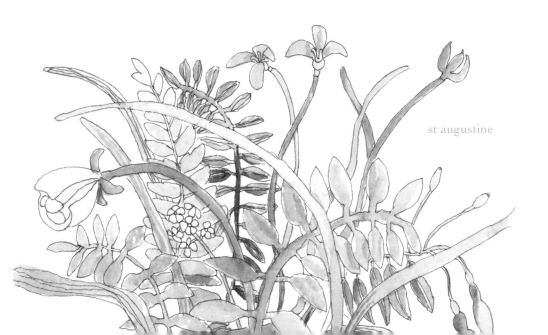

st augustine

sadness flies away
on the wings of time

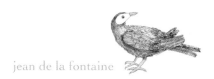

jean de la fontaine

when you ask
the answer
shall be given

rumi

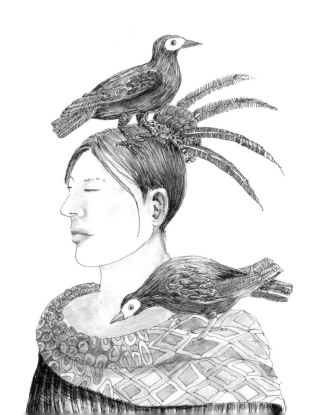

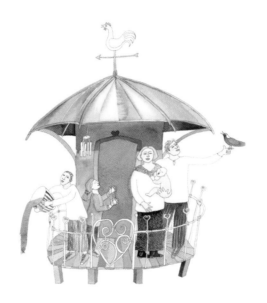

he who kisses the joy as it flies lives in eternity's sunrise

william blake

when it is
dark enough
you can see
the stars

ralph waldo emerson

learn silence
from the talkative
tolerance
from the intolerant
and kindness
from the unkind

be grateful to those teachers

kahlil gibran

do not cry
because it is over

smile
because it happened

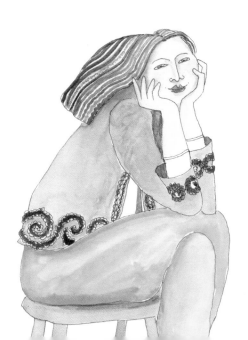

you are

since everybody is an individual
nobody can be you

you are unique

no one can tell you how to use your time
it is yours
your life is your own
you mold it
you make it

eleanor roosevelt

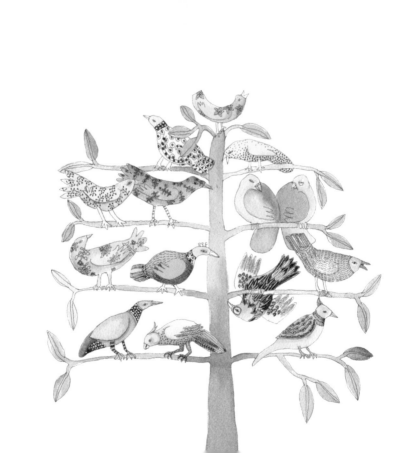

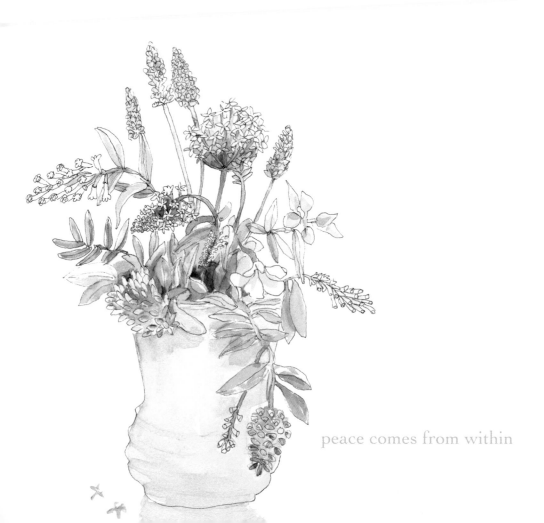

peace comes from within

hope well
and
have well

words
have
wings

speak
good
things

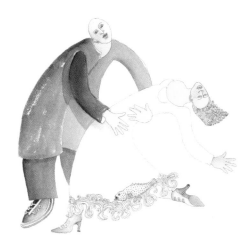

be like the flower
turn your face to the sun

kahlil gibran

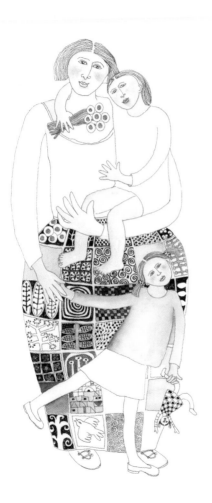

look for the answer
inside your question

rumi

look for

put your ear down
close to your soul
and listen hard

anne sexton

the answer

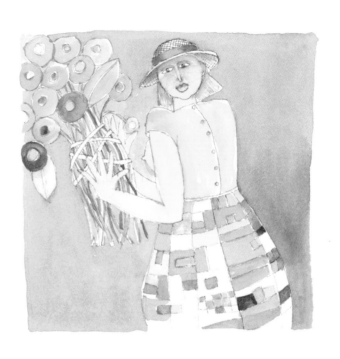

act mindfully

accept entirely

move strongly

think softly

speak beautifully

live simply

love completely

i saw grief
drinking a cup of sorrow
and called out
"it tastes sweet does it not?"

"you've caught me"
grief answered
"and you've ruined my business
how can i sell sorrow
when you know it's a blessing?"

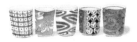

rumi

people touch our lives
if only for a moment
and yet we're not the same
from that moment on

the time is not important
the moment is forever

fern bork

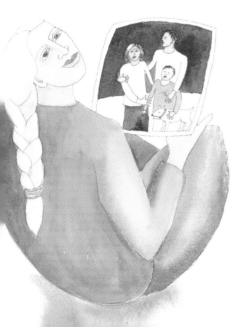

beyond ideas
there is a field

will you meet me there?

rumi

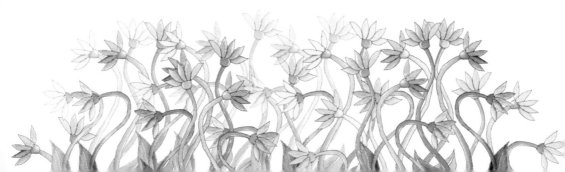

there comes a time
when sea and land come to rest

there comes a time when even the heavens withdraw

there comes a time when weary travelers
need a rest from the journey

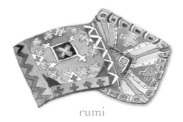

rumi

on these sands
and in the clefts of the rocks
in the depths of the sea
in the creaking of the pines
you'll spy secret footprints
and catch far-off voices
from the homecoming celebration

homer

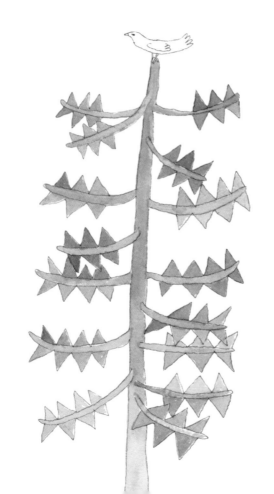

there are things that we don't want to happen
but have to accept

things we don't want to know
but have to learn

and people we can't live without
but have to let go

this is love

to fly toward a secret sky
to cause a hundred veils
to fall each moment

first to let go of life

finally
to take a step without feet

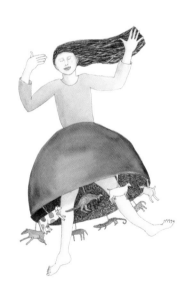

rumi

nothing beautiful in this world
is ever really lost

all things beloved
live on in our hearts forever

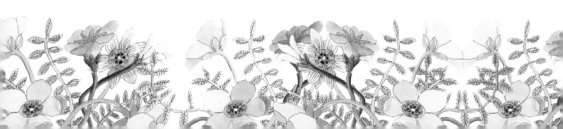

seek for the resting place
not in the earth

but in the hearts of many

rumi

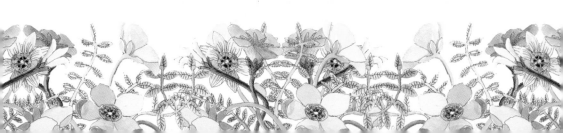

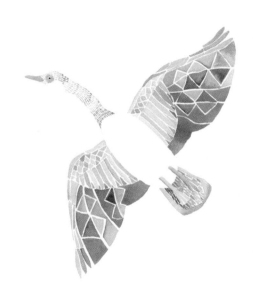

how do geese know when to fly to the sun?
who tells them the seasons?
how do we humans know
when it is time to move on?
how do we know when to go?

as with the migrant birds
so surely with us
there is a voice within
if only we would listen to it
that tells us so certainly
when to go forth
into the unknown

elisabeth kübler-ross

when we have done all the work
we were sent to earth to do
we are allowed to shed our body
which imprisons our soul
like a cocoon encloses
the future butterfly
and when the time is right
we can let go of it
and we will be free of pain
free of fears and worries
free as a very beautiful butterfly
returning home to God

which is a place where we are never alone
where we continue to grow
to sing
and to dance
where we are with those we loved
and where we are surrounded
with more love
than we can ever imagine

from a letter to a child with cancer
elisabeth kübler-ross

there are no mistakes
no coincidences

all events are blessings
given to us
to learn from

elisabeth kübler-ross

yes there is a nirvana

it is in leading your sheep to a green pasture
and in putting your child to sleep
and in writing the last line of your poem

kahlil gibran

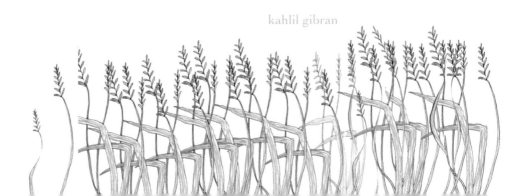

light the

path

to love

let us fall in love again
and scatter gold dust all over the world

let us become a new spring
and feel the breeze drift in the heaven's scent

let us dress the earth in green
and like the sap of a young tree
let the grace from within sustain us

let us carve gems out of our stony hearts
and let them light the path to love

the glance of love is crystal clear
and we are blessed by its light

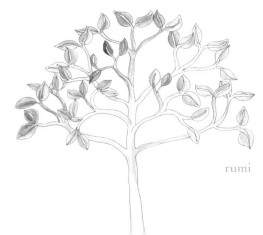

rumi

if in the twilight of memory
we should meet once more

we shall speak again together
and you shall sing to me a deeper song

and if our hands should meet
in another dream

we shall build
another tower in the sky

kahlil gibran

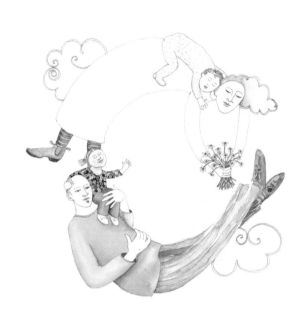